PROSTATE CANCER DIET COOKBOOK:

FOR NEWLY DIAGNOSED

Complete Beginner Procedures On Food Recipes, Guided Meal Plans, And Healthy Lifestyle Tips To Manage, Strive, And Live Well With Prostate Cancer

DR. EMMY BROOKS

ABOUT THIS BOOK

In the realm of health and wellness manuals, the "Prostate Cancer Diet Cookbook" stands as a beacon of knowledge and empowerment. The introductory chapters pave the way for a profound understanding of the intricate relationship between prostate health and nutrition. The authors skillfully navigate through the basics of prostate cancer, shedding light on risk factors and prevention strategies, while underscoring the paramount importance of early detection.

A highlight of this culinary guide lies in its exploration of the pivotal role nutrition plays in preventing and managing prostate cancer. The book offers a comprehensive look at essential nutrients for prostate health, presenting a roadmap for crafting a balanced and nutritious diet. It not only identifies foods to include for optimal well-being but also advises on those to avoid, providing readers with practical tools to make informed dietary choices.

Further enhancing its value, the cookbook delves into the creation of a prostate-friendly pantry, offering insights into stocking up on essential ingredients, selecting the right oils and fats, and incorporating whole grains and legumes. This meticulous attention to detail extends to a spotlight on prostate-boosting superfoods, accompanied by easy-to-follow recipes that seamlessly integrate these nutritional powerhouses into everyday meals.

A notable feature of the "Prostate Cancer Diet Cookbook" is its emphasis on practicality, demonstrated through meal prep tips that save time, batch cooking strategies for efficiency, and the assurance of a variety of flavors in every dish. The recipes provided for breakfast, lunch, and dinner are not only delicious but also specifically designed to promote prostate health, with a focus on balancing macronutrients and micronutrients.

Moreover, the book extends its reach to lifestyle factors, acknowledging the importance of hydration, physical activity, stress management, and adequate sleep in maintaining prostate health. It goes beyond being a mere cookbook, transforming into a holistic guide for those seeking sustained well-being through long-term strategies, regular check-ups, and a celebration of successes in the journey toward prostate health. The "Prostate Cancer Diet Cookbook" is a treasure trove of knowledge, offering readers a practical and elevating approach to enhancing their overall well-being.

DISCLAIMER

This book's content is solely intended for general informative purposes. About the availability, applicability, correctness, completeness, and trustworthiness of the data or recipes in this book, the author provides no guarantees of any sort, either stated or implied. You bear full responsibility for any reliance you may have on such material.

The advice, diagnosis, or treatment provided by a qualified medical expert is not to be replaced by this cookbook. When in doubt about a medical problem, never hesitate to consult your doctor or another trained healthcare professional. Never ignore medical advice from professionals or put off getting it because of something you've read in this book.

At the time of publishing, the author of this book has taken reasonable steps to guarantee that the information is correct and current. He does not, however, guarantee that the data will be error-free or that it will satisfy any certain performance or quality standards. Any negative repercussions that may arise from using or applying the material in this book are not the responsibility of the author, publisher, or distributor.

In this book, references or mentions of individuals, products, websites, organizations, or other names are for informational purposes only and do not imply endorsement or affiliation with the author. The author has no control over the nature, content, and availability of referenced or mentioned entities. Any reliance on such information is at the reader's own risk.

The inclusion of any references does not necessarily imply a recommendation or endorse the views expressed within them. The author or publisher shall not be liable for any loss or damage arising out of or in connection with, the use of this book.

INTRODUCTION

UNDERSTANDING PROSTATE CANCER AND NUTRITION

Brief Overview of Prostate Cancer:

Prostate cancer is a prevalent form of cancer that occurs in the prostate, a small walnut-shaped gland in men that produces seminal fluid. It is essential to understand the basics of prostate cancer to make informed decisions about your health.

Prostate cancer often progresses slowly and may not cause noticeable symptoms in its early stages. However, as it advances, it can lead to serious health issues. Factors such as age, family history, and race can influence the risk of developing prostate cancer.

Detecting prostate cancer in its early stages significantly improves the chances of successful treatment. Regular screenings, including prostate-specific antigen (PSA) tests and digital rectal exams, are crucial for early detection.

It is important for individuals, especially men over the age of 50, to be proactive about their health and discuss screening options with their healthcare providers.

Understanding the characteristics of prostate cancer, its risk factors, and the available screening methods lays the foundation for making informed decisions about preventive measures and potential dietary interventions to support prostate health.

The Impact of Diet on Prostate Health:

Diet plays a crucial role in overall health, and its impact on prostate health is no exception. Numerous studies suggest a strong connection between diet and the risk of developing prostate cancer. While no single food or nutrient can guarantee protection against prostate cancer, adopting a prostate-friendly diet may contribute to reducing the risk and supporting overall well-being.

There is evidence linking the ingestion of specific foods and nutrients to a decreased risk of prostate cancer. Berries, tomatoes, and broccoli are examples of fruits and vegetables high in antioxidants.

These foods also include substances that may help reduce inflammation and oxidative stress, which may help maintain a healthy prostate. Furthermore, studies have suggested that omega-3 fatty acids, which are present in walnuts, flaxseeds, and fatty fish, may help lower the risk of prostate cancer.

 Conversely, it could be wise to reduce your consumption of red and processed meats, high-fat dairy products, and excessive calcium. A higher risk of prostate cancer has been associated with several dietary patterns.

Comprehending these dietary correlations enables people to make knowledgeable food selections and take a proactive stance toward prostate health via diet.

The Value of a Nutritious and Balanced Diet

Eating a healthy, well-balanced diet is essential for good health in general and for prostate health in particular. A well-balanced diet supports cellular health and strengthens the immune system by giving the body the vital vitamins, minerals, and nutrients it needs to perform at its best. Adopting a diet high in fruits, vegetables, whole grains, and lean proteins can be a fundamental step in promoting prostate health for people who are worried about prostate cancer.

Drinking enough water is another essential component of a healthy diet. Maintaining adequate hydration aids in the removal of waste products and toxins from the body, which can help reduce inflammation and other health problems. Drinking herbal teas and eating plenty of fruits and vegetables will help you stay properly hydrated throughout the day.

Portion control is essential in addition to choosing certain foods. Retaining a healthy weight lowers the chance of getting prostate cancer among other malignancies. Physical exercise and calorie intake balance promote healthy weight management.

People are empowered to make educated decisions while choosing and cooking meals when they are aware of nutrition labels, portion sizes, hidden sugars, and bad fats.

Adopting a healthy, well-balanced diet promotes longevity and general well-being in addition to prostate health.

CHAPTER ONE

PROSTATE CANCER FUNDAMENTALS

Prostate cancer: What Is It?

One kind of cancer that arises in the prostate is prostate cancer. The prostate is a tiny gland situated in front of the rectum and beneath the bladder. The prostate, which generates seminal fluid that nourishes and transports sperm, is an essential component of the male reproductive system. Uncontrolled growth of prostate cells can result in the formation of a tumor, which may be malignant.

Men and others close to them must understand the fundamentals of prostate cancer. Prostate cancer often progresses slowly, and many men may not exhibit any signs while the disease is first developing. But when the illness worsens, it may result in discomfort, urination issues, and other symptoms.

It is critical to take preventative action and to be aware of the risk factors linked to prostate cancer.

Risk Elements and Preventive Techniques

Prostate cancer can arise from a variety of causes, and prevention requires knowledge of these risks. Among the risk variables that cannot be changed are age, race, and family history. Men are more likely to get prostate cancer as they become older, and most instances affect those over 65. Prostate cancer risk also increases if a close relative, like a father or brother, has had the disease. Compared to males from other ethnic backgrounds, African-American men are more likely to develop prostate cancer.

Although certain risk factors are unavoidable, adopting certain lifestyle choices and implementing preventive measures can greatly lower the likelihood of acquiring prostate cancer. Three essential elements of a prostate cancer prevention plan include avoiding tobacco products, exercising regularly, and maintaining a healthy diet.

Including particular items in your diet that have been demonstrated to have preventive effects against prostate cancer can also be a proactive and successful approach.

The Value of Early Identification

Prostate cancer treatment is most successful when it is detected early. Digital rectal exams (DRE) and blood testing for the prostate-specific antigen (PSA) are two important diagnostics that are essential for spotting possible problems early on. Early detection of prostate cancer increases the likelihood of successful results and often leads to more effective treatment options.

Men should be aware of the telltale signs and symptoms of prostate cancer, which include changes in urination, pain when urinating, and blood in the urine. A healthcare provider's routine examinations can assist in identifying and evaluating any possible dangers. Men need to take an active role in their health and talk to their doctors about any concerns they may have.

Raising people's knowledge of the value of early detection can give them the confidence to take charge of their health and get help as soon as possible.

 To sum up, a thorough approach to prostate health must include knowledge of what prostate cancer is, identification of risk factors, use of preventive measures, and stressing the significance of early detection. Through early detection and intervention, individuals can greatly lower their chance of getting prostate cancer and raise the likelihood of positive outcomes by embracing a proactive approach and incorporating healthy practices into their lifestyle.

CHAPTER TWO

DIET AND HEALTH OF THE PROSTATE
Nutrition's Part in Prostate Cancer Management and Prevention:

Maintaining optimal health requires an understanding of the critical role that nutrition plays in both preventing and controlling prostate cancer. A prostate-friendly diet can dramatically lower the risk of acquiring prostate cancer, which is the second most frequent cancer among men worldwide.

First and foremost, it's critical to concentrate on eating a diet high in antioxidants because these compounds are critical in counteracting dangerous free radicals that may aid in the growth of cancer cells. A wide variety of antioxidants can be included by including colored fruits and vegetables, such as cruciferous vegetables, tomatoes, and berries. These foods specifically target prostate health in addition to supporting general health.

Furthermore, it is essential to keep a balanced diet that includes the right amounts of complex carbs, lean proteins, and healthy fats. Flaxseeds and fatty fish, such as salmon, are rich sources of omega-3 fatty acids, which have anti-inflammatory qualities that may benefit prostate health. Consuming enough fiber from fruits, vegetables, and whole grains facilitates digestion and helps control hormones associated with prostate cancer.

Because processed foods, sugary snacks, and red or processed meats have been linked to an elevated risk of prostate cancer, it is equally vital to limit your intake of these foods. Reducing your intake of saturated fats, which are frequently found in fried foods and high-fat dairy products, is advised since too much of them can be harmful to your prostate.

Prostate cancer risk may be decreased by taking a proactive approach to nutrition, such as choosing a Mediterranean-style diet high in fruits, vegetables, whole grains, and healthy fats. This dietary pattern offers a pleasant and comprehensive approach to prostate health maintenance by emphasizing the consumption of almonds, salmon, and olive oil.

Vital Elements for Healthy Prostate Function:

To keep your prostate functioning at its best, you must make sure you are getting enough of the necessary nutrients. An essential mineral that is critical to prostate health is zinc. Zinc-rich foods include lean meats, pumpkin seeds, and oysters. Brazil nuts, sunflower seeds, and whole grains include selenium, another essential element with antioxidant qualities that support prostate health in general.

Prostate health depends on vitamin D because it modulates immunological response and cell proliferation. While exposure to sunlight is a natural source of vitamin D, diets rich in foods such as egg yolks, dairy products with added fortification, and fatty fish are also beneficial. Nuts, seeds, and green leafy vegetables are good sources of vitamin E, a powerful antioxidant that offers additional defense against oxidative stress.

Tomatoes, watermelon, and pink grapefruit are good sources of lycopene, a carotenoid that has been associated with a lower risk of prostate cancer. Not only do these meals enhance flavor, but they also strengthen the body's defenses against problems associated with the prostate.

Though sometimes forgotten, maintaining adequate hydration is essential to prostate health. Water promotes a healthy prostate by supporting general body functioning and aiding in the removal of pollutants from the body. Antioxidant-rich green tea is an additional great beverage option that may shield prostate cells.

Foods to Take and Leave Out:

Including some foods and avoiding others while creating a diet plan for prostate cancer are essential measures in preserving good prostate health. A range of vitamins, minerals, and antioxidants are provided by a variety of fruits and vegetables, therefore it is imperative to include them in your diet. Broccoli, tomatoes, bell peppers, and berries are very good for prostate health.

Lean protein sources like fish, chicken, and lentils help maintain muscle mass without having the possible side effects of processed and red meat. Omega-3 fatty acids, which are abundant in fatty fish like salmon and mackerel and have anti-inflammatory qualities, support prostate health.

Nuts and seeds, including walnuts, flaxseeds, and almonds, are great providers of important minerals including vitamin E, zinc, and selenium. These wholesome snacks not only satisfy hunger but also promote prostate health.

Yet, since red and processed meats have been linked to a higher risk of prostate cancer, it is crucial to restrict your intake of these foods. Dairy products with high-fat content should be consumed in moderation; whenever possible, choose plant-based or low-fat alternatives.

Limiting processed and sugary foods—including snacks and desserts—is advised since they aggravate inflammation and may have detrimental effects on the health of the prostate.

 As a result, implementing a prostate cancer diet requires choosing foods that are high in nutrients and actively promote general health. Proactively managing one's prostate health can help prevent prostate cancer and promote long-term wellness by prioritizing a wide variety of fruits, vegetables, lean proteins, and important nutrients.

CHAPTER THREE

BUILDING A PROSTATE-FRIENDLY PANTRY
Keeping up with Necessary Ingredients:

Putting together a pantry that is prostate-friendly starts with acquiring staples that support a healthy, well-balanced diet. Choosing foods high in antioxidants, vitamins, and minerals is part of this process; these nutrients are essential for prostate health. Fresh fruits and vegetables should come first because they are high in antioxidant-rich vitamins C and E. Broccoli, leafy greens, citrus fruits, and berries can all be great foods to include in your diet.

You should also keep lean proteins as a regular in your cupboard. Go for foods like fish, tofu, skinless chicken, and beans. These high-protein choices include the essential amino acids without the added saturated fats often seen in red meats.

Additionally, because of their omega-3 fatty acids, which have been connected to prostate health, nuts and seeds like walnuts and flaxseeds can be advantageous.

Add tomatoes and tomato-based products to your diet since they are rich in lycopene, a powerful antioxidant linked to prostate health. Think of tomato paste, tomato sauce, and canned tomatoes as handy pantry staples. For flavorful soups and stews, use low-sodium vegetable or chicken broth as the basis without sacrificing health.

Another key item in a pantry that is prostate-friendly is whole grains. Whole wheat pasta, quinoa, and brown rice are all great options because they include a range of minerals and fiber. For the most nutritional impact, choose whole grains over refined ones.

Give low-fat or fat-free choices priority in the dairy area. Stock your pantry with Greek yogurt, skim milk, and low-fat cheese to get your calcium fix without going overboard on saturated fat.

Selecting the Proper Fats and Oils:

Making the proper oil and fat choices is essential for prostate health. Choose oils high in mono- and polyunsaturated fats as they are heart-healthy. For instance, olive oil is a great option because of its high monounsaturated fat content and possible anti-inflammatory qualities.

Omega-3 fatty acid-rich flaxseed oil is a useful addition to any pantry. These fatty acids are simply added to smoothies or salad dressings and have been linked to prostate health.

Despite its popularity, coconut oil should only be used sparingly because of its high saturated fat content. Use it sparingly for some dishes instead, or choose avocado oil as a substitute, which offers a comparable richness without raising issues with saturated fat.

Use cooking sprays or a modest amount of heart-healthy oils when choosing fats for cooking.

Cooking techniques like baking, grilling, or steaming reduce the need for additional fat and maintain the nutritious value of your food.

Using Complete Grains and Legumes:

A prostate-friendly diet's mainstays include whole grains and legumes, which offer fiber, vital nutrients, and plant-based proteins. Start by stocking your cupboard with nutritious grains, such as quinoa, brown rice, oats, and whole wheat products. Because of their high fiber content, these grains support healthy digestion and general well-being.

Legumes are a great source of fiber and plant-based protein. This includes beans, lentils, and chickpeas. You can choose dried or canned choices, but be aware that canned ones have more sodium. Before adding canned legumes to your meals, give them a quick rinse under water to cut down on sodium.

To find a nutrient-dense substitute for conventionally refined pasta, try experimenting with several kinds of whole-grain and legume-based pasta. These types make a filling foundation for a variety of recipes and frequently have a greater fiber level.

To get the most nutritious value out of whole grains and legumes, try blending them in salads or grain bowls. It is simpler for beginners to embrace and stick to these dietary modifications when these essentials are incorporated gradually into your diet, as this facilitates a smooth transition to a prostate-friendly lifestyle.

CHAPTER FOUR

SUPERFOODS THAT BOOST PROSTATE
Emphasizing Superfoods for Healthy Prostate Functions:

Prostate health is essential to overall well-being, and maintaining a healthy prostate can be greatly aided by including superfoods that stimulate the prostate in your diet. These superfoods are abundant in minerals, antioxidants, and other substances that support prostate health and may even help prevent conditions related to the prostate, such as prostate cancer.

Tomatoes are an exceptional superfood for prostate health. Lycopene, a potent antioxidant found in tomatoes, has been linked to a decreased risk of prostate cancer. Cooking tomatoes increases the body's absorption of lycopene, thus tomato-based sauces, soups, and stews are great options. Tomatoes add flavor to a variety of meals and are a delightful and easy addition to any diet.

Green tea is another superfood to take into account. Green tea, which is rich in catechins, which are antioxidants, has been researched for its ability to lower the incidence of prostate cancer.

Adding green tea as a drink substitute is an easy way to integrate this superfood into your daily routine. It can be consumed hot or cold, and you can customize it to your preference by adding honey or a squeeze of lemon.

Broccoli, cauliflower, and Brussels sprouts are examples of cruciferous vegetables, which are also superfoods that support the prostate. Sulforaphane, a substance found in these veggies, has demonstrated the potential to inhibit and delay the growth of prostate cancer cells.

Try roasting or steaming these veggies as a side dish or adding them to salads for a crisp and nutrient-dense twist to incorporate them into your diet.

Easy Ways to Add Superfoods That Boost the Prostate to Your Diet:

It's not difficult to include prostate-boosting superfoods in your regular diet. It can be accomplished by taking easy, pleasurable actions that eventually become a routine. Over time, little adjustments made at first can have a big impact.

Making a weekly meal plan with a range of superfoods is one simple way. For example, base your meals on tomatoes and use them in salads, sandwiches, and sauces. Try experimenting with different tomato types, like heirlooms or cherry tomatoes, to give your meals a variety of tastes and textures.

Investigating novel recipes that incorporate green tea is an additional strategy. Green tea can be integrated into sauces and dressings, added to smoothies, and used in meat marinades. When you add the essence of green tea to other foods, you improve their taste and nutritional value.

Think of inventive ways to include cruciferous veggies in your favorite recipes. For a healthier twist, try roasting Brussels sprouts with a sprinkle of olive oil and your preferred spices, blending broccoli into a creamy soup, or making a cauliflower-based pizza crust. You can facilitate a smooth and joyful transition by including these superfoods in well-known meals.

Recipes Featuring Prostate-Boosting Super Foods:

To make the process of incorporating prostate-boosting super foods even more accessible, here are two delicious and easy-to-follow recipes that highlight the benefits of tomatoes and cruciferous vegetables:

1. Lycopene-Rich Tomato Basil Pasta:

Ingredients:

- Whole wheat or gluten-free pasta

- Fresh tomatoes or canned crushed tomatoes

- Fresh basil leaves

- Garlic cloves, minced

- Olive oil

- Salt and pepper to taste

- Grated Parmesan cheese (optional)

Instructions:

1. Cook the pasta according to package instructions.

2. In a pan, sauté minced garlic in olive oil until fragrant.

3. Add fresh tomatoes or canned crushed tomatoes to the pan and simmer until the sauce thickens.

4. Stir in chopped fresh basil and season with salt and pepper.

5. Toss the cooked pasta in the tomato basil sauce until well coated.

6.   Optional: Sprinkle with grated Parmesan cheese before serving.

2. Roasted Garlic and Parmesan Brussels Sprouts:

Ingredients:

- Brussels sprouts, halved

- Olive oil

- Minced garlic

- Grated Parmesan cheese

- Salt and pepper to taste

Instructions:

1.   Set oven temperature to 400°F, or 200°C.

2.   Toss halved Brussels sprouts with olive oil, minced garlic, salt, and pepper.

3.   Spread the Brussels sprouts on a baking sheet in a single layer.

4.   Roast in the preheated oven for 20-25 minutes or until golden brown and crispy.

5.   Sprinkle grated Parmesan cheese over the roasted Brussels sprouts before serving.

These recipes not only showcase the prostate-boosting superfoods but also demonstrate how simple it is to incorporate them into your daily meals. By enjoying these flavorful dishes regularly, you'll be actively contributing to the health of your prostate in a tasty and satisfying way.

3. Green Tea-Marinated Grilled Salmon:

Ingredients:

- Salmon fillets

- Green tea bags

- Soy sauce

- Honey

- Ginger, minced

- Garlic cloves, minced

- Sesame oil

- Lemon wedges for garnish

Instructions:

1.   Brew a strong cup of green tea using two tea bags. Let it cool.

2.   In a bowl, mix the cooled green tea, soy sauce, honey, minced ginger, minced garlic, and a dash of sesame oil to create the marinade.

3.   Place salmon fillets in a shallow dish and pour the marinade over them. Marinate for at least 30 minutes.

4.   Preheat the grill and cook the salmon for 4-5 minutes per side or until cooked through.

5.   Serve the grilled salmon with lemon wedges for a zesty touch.

4. Quinoa Salad with Roasted Broccoli and Cauliflower:

Ingredients:

- Quinoa, cooked

- Broccoli florets

- Cauliflower florets

- Cherry tomatoes, halved

- Red onion, finely chopped

- Feta cheese, crumbled

- Olive oil

- Balsamic vinegar

- Salt and pepper to taste

Instructions:

1. Set oven temperature to 400°F, or 200°C.

2. Toss broccoli and cauliflower florets with olive oil, salt, and pepper, then roast for 20-25 minutes until golden brown.

3. In a large bowl, combine cooked quinoa, roasted broccoli, roasted cauliflower, cherry tomatoes, red onion, and crumbled feta cheese.

4. Drizzle with olive oil and balsamic vinegar. Toss gently to combine.

5. Adjust salt and pepper to taste and serve chilled.

5. Tomato and Avocado Salsa:

Ingredients:

- Ripe tomatoes, diced

- Avocado, diced

- Red onion, finely chopped

- Fresh cilantro, chopped

- Lime juice

- Jalapeño, minced (optional for heat)

- To taste, add salt and pepper

- Whole-grain tortilla chips for serving

Instructions:

1. In a bowl, combine diced tomatoes, diced avocado, chopped red onion, and fresh cilantro.

2. Squeeze lime juice over the mixture and add minced jalapeño if you desire some heat.

3. Gently toss the ingredients until well combined.

4. To taste, add salt and pepper for seasoning.

5.   Allow the salsa to sit for 10-15 minutes to let the flavors meld. Serve with whole-grain tortilla chips for a refreshing and prostate-healthy snack.

Enjoying these meals regularly not only contributes to prostate health but also adds variety and excitement to your culinary repertoire.

CHAPTER FIVE

THE PROSTATE CANCER DIET PLAN

Creating a Personalized Diet Plan:

Starting a food plan tailored to prostate cancer demands careful planning and individual attention. A beginner should start by being aware of their unique lifestyle, preferences, and health concerns. It can be very helpful to speak with a medical practitioner or a registered dietician with expertise in cancer. These professionals can evaluate the patient's past medical history, the present state of health, and any possible dietary limitations.

Finding foods that are high in antioxidants, vitamins, and minerals that are proven to enhance prostate health is the first step. This involves including foods high in antioxidants, such as leafy greens, broccoli, tomatoes, and berries, into your diet. These foods also contain phytochemicals that fight cancer.

Incorporating whole grains, lean proteins, and healthy fats into the meal plan is vital to provide a comprehensive and balanced base.

To make sure that the body gets a wide range of vital nutrients, it is imperative to concentrate on eating a varied and nutrient-dense array of foods. This customized strategy ensures that the diet is both enjoyable for long-term adherence and health promotion by taking into account each person's taste preferences and making adjustments accordingly.

Keeping Micronutrients and Macronutrients in Balance:

An efficient diet plan for prostate cancer must balance macronutrients (proteins, fats, and carbohydrates) with micronutrients (vitamins and minerals). A beginner should be aware of the importance of every nutritional category and how it affects general health.

Lean meats, lentils, and dairy products are good sources of protein, which is needed for immunological response and cell repair. Nuts, avocados, and olive oil are good sources of healthy fats that help reduce inflammation. Carbohydrates—especially those from fruits and whole grains—provide the fiber and energy needed for a healthy digestive system.

Micronutrients with prostate-protective qualities include zinc, vitamin D, and selenium. Nuts, seeds, fatty fish, and whole grains are good providers of these vital micronutrients. A beginner should strive to have these nutrients distributed evenly throughout each meal, making sure that no one group is overemphasized.

Portion management is just as important as variation. Keeping an eye on portion sizes promotes weight control, helps avoid overindulgence, and guarantees that the body gets the proper ratio of nutrients without needless excess.

Timing of Meals and Portion Management:

Optimizing the efficacy of a prostate cancer diet plan requires an understanding of the importance of meal timing and portion control. When it comes to meal scheduling, a beginner should emphasize regularity and consistency. Creating a schedule that consists of three main meals as well as snacks will help you stay energetic all day.

Every meal has to be nutritionally balanced, with a variety of healthy fats, proteins, and carbs. This distribution facilitates improved nutrient absorption in addition to promoting general wellness. A beginner can start by adding whole grains, lean proteins, and vibrant veggies to their meals to make a dish that is both aesthetically pleasing and full of nutrients.

Using smaller plates and bowls might be a useful method to improve portion control. A newbie will find it easier to control their intake as a result of the visually reduced portion sizes. It's also critical to pay attention to your body's internal signals of hunger and fullness. The body can communicate when it is full when you eat slowly and enjoy every bite, which helps you avoid overindulging.

The strategy may include snacks in between meals, but it's crucial to pick nutrient-dense foods like fruits, almonds, or yogurt.

This keeps energy levels stable and inhibits overindulgence in hunger, which can result in bad eating decisions.

These doable actions can help a beginner understand the intricacies of portion management and meal time, which will ultimately make the execution of a prostate cancer diet plan more feasible and sustainable.

CHAPTER SIX

USEFUL TIPS FOR PREPARING MEALS
Quick and Easy Ways to Prepare Meals:

When it comes to meal preparation, efficiency is crucial, particularly for those on a diet for prostate cancer. Start by organizing your meals for the coming week to save time and streamline the process. Make sure to include breakfast, lunch, supper, and snacks in your comprehensive menu. Make a thorough shopping list by listing all of the materials required for each recipe.

Invest in top-notch food storage containers to maintain the freshness and readiness of your goods. This will prolong the shelf life of your products and facilitate grab-and-go meals throughout the workweek. Additionally, think about portioning out cereals, marinating proteins, and washing and slicing veggies ahead of time.

In this manner, you may concentrate on assembling your meals when it's time to cook instead of wasting valuable time on preparation.

Additionally, select recipes that facilitate multitasking. For example, you can roast veggies in the oven at the same time as a soup simmers on the stove. This method makes the most of the time you spend in the kitchen and guarantees that you always have a range of ingredients on hand for a variety of meals that you may prepare throughout the week.

Set aside particular days to prepare your meals to further simplify the cooking procedure. Many people find that setting aside a few hours on Sunday to get ready for the following week works well. In addition to saving time on hectic workdays, this promotes diet consistency for prostate cancer.

Cooking in Bulk for Optimal Efficiency:

For those looking to prepare meals more efficiently, batch cooking is revolutionary. The idea is to prepare bigger amounts of food at once so you have ready-made ingredients for several meals. Because it makes meal prep easier, this method is especially helpful for inexperienced cooks.

Start by choosing recipes that work well for large quantities of cooking. Grain-based salads, casseroles, and stews are great examples of dishes. After deciding on your recipes, gather all the components and adjust the amounts by double or triplicate. This will ensure that you have enough portions for the entire week in addition to saving you time.

To handle greater numbers, invest in sizable baking sheets, cooking pots, and storage containers. When preparing proteins in large quantities for freezing, think about marinating them first and then splitting them into smaller parts. This will cut down on the amount of time you spend preparing meals every day because you can just defrost and use them as needed.

Keeping track of your batch-cooked foods requires labeling. Indicate on each container exactly what is inside and when it was prepared.

This guarantees that you eat meals at their peak freshness and also aids in maintaining organization.

To ease yourself into batch cooking as a novice, start with one or two dishes. You'll grow accustomed to this effective strategy over time, which will make sticking to your prostate cancer diet easier.

Making Sure Your Meals Have a Range of Flavors:

It's crucial to keep your meals varied in flavor to ensure nutritional balance and satisfaction. Investigate various herbs, spices, and seasonings to improve the flavor of your food without sacrificing health when following a prostate cancer diet.

Make sure your spice rack is stocked first. Add basic spices like turmeric, coriander, cumin, onion powder, and garlic powder. These spices can improve your health in addition to giving your food more dimension. Try experimenting with herbs such as rosemary, thyme, and basil to improve the flavor of your food as a whole.

Another approach to make sure your meals are varied is to include a variety of textures. For example, to add texture to a batch-cooked quinoa salad, try adding some crunchy nuts or seeds on top. Vegetables that have been roasted or grilled can also offer a delightful contrast to softer ingredients.

Without using a lot of salt or bad fats, citrus fruits like lemons and limes can be great flavor enhancers. To brighten and give a burst of freshness to salads, grilled proteins, or roasted veggies, squeeze fresh lemon juice over them.

Additionally, experimenting with various cooking methods can help create a wide range of flavors. Different cooking methods, such as grilling, roasting, steaming, and sautéing, give food unique flavors. To keep your taste interested, mix up your meal prep techniques by utilizing a range of these techniques.

If you're a beginner, begin by adding one or two new herbs or spices to your meals every week. With time, you'll gain self-assurance in mixing flavors and preparing a wide variety of dishes that please your palate and follow your prostate cancer diet.

CHAPTER SEVEN

SCRUMPTIOUS AND HEALTHFUL MORNING RECIPES

Simple Recipes for Prostate-Friendly Breakfasts:

Making a breakfast that is prostate-friendly doesn't have to be difficult; in fact, simplicity sometimes works best. Take into consideration options such as a vegetable omelet for a quick and nourishing breakfast. In a nonstick skillet, start by sautéing onions, bell peppers, and spinach with a small amount of olive oil. After beating the eggs, cover the veggies with them and heat until the eggs are set. Add a pinch of turmeric, a spice that has been shown to have anti-inflammatory effects and improve prostate health.

A yogurt parfait with toppings that are prostate-friendly is another simple breakfast option. Start with low-fat or Greek yogurt and top with a range of antioxidant-rich fruits, like berries.

Finish with a small handful of nuts, such as walnuts, which are well-known for their omega-3 fatty acids, which promote prostate health in general.

Including Protein, Whole Grains, and Fruits:

Prostate health requires a balanced breakfast, which can be made tasty and nourishing by including a variety of fruits, complete grains, and proteins. Choose a whole grain toast with avocado slices on top. Avocados are rich in healthy lipids that support prostate health in addition to being creamy and filling. For a dose of vitamin C, which is thought to have preventive properties against prostate cancer, pair it with a side of fresh grapefruit.

If you'd rather have a heartier breakfast, think about making quinoa bowls. Whole grains like quinoa are an excellent source of fiber and protein. Once the quinoa is cooked as directed on the package, add sliced tomatoes, cucumbers, and lean protein, like tofu or grilled chicken.

Use herbs such as cilantro or parsley to season food for flavor and prostate-healthy properties.

Smoothies In The Morning And Options For Energy:

Smoothies are a great way to get a nutritional boost in the morning. Blend spinach, berries, banana, and protein powder for a prostate-friendly smoothie. Berries provide antioxidants to the mixture, while spinach gives a healthy dose of folate. Inherently sweet and high in potassium, bananas are good for the general health of the prostate. Pick a protein powder—vegetable or whey—that fits your nutritional requirements.

A green tea smoothie is a great alternative if you're searching for something invigorating. After brewing and cooling, combine frozen mango, pineapple, and a small handful of kale with your brewed green tea. Antioxidants found in green tea, along with the blend of fruits and vegetables, make for a revitalizing and refreshing start to the day.

Including these simple, well-balanced breakfast options made with prostate-friendly ingredients will allow you to have a wonderful morning routine that promotes overall health.

CHAPTER EIGHT

HEALTHFUL LUNCH SUGGESTIONS

Efficient and Filling Lunch Recipes:

Making easy yet filling lunch recipes is crucial to keeping a prostate cancer-friendly diet in place since they guarantee a healthy, well-balanced meal. Simplifying recipes is essential for first-time cooks, and using readily available items is a terrific place to start.

A simple recipe worth trying is a quinoa salad with vibrant greens. Grain rich in protein, quinoa makes a great foundation. Start by giving the quinoa a thorough rinse and cooking it as directed on the package. Chop several veggies, including bell peppers, cucumbers, and cherry tomatoes, while the quinoa is cooking. Combine the cooked quinoa with these colorful veggies and toss with a simple vinaigrette of lemon juice, olive oil, and a dash of salt.

Antioxidants and fiber give this light salad a powerful nutritional boost in addition to being easy to make.

A lean protein whole grain wrap is another quick alternative. Pick a whole grain tortilla and stuff it with turkey grilled chicken, or any other lean protein source. For a healthier take on mayonnaise, top with sliced avocado, a hefty portion of leafy greens, and a dollop of Greek yogurt. In addition to being tasty, this protein-rich wrap meets the requirements of a prostate cancer diet by offering vital nutrients.

Including Lean Proteins and Vegetables:

Including veggies and lean meats is important when it comes to a diet for prostate cancer. This approach can be made simpler for beginners by concentrating on nutrient-dense, colorful selections that are easily found at nearby grocery stores.

Try a roasted vegetable medley for a veggie-rich lunch that's easy even for beginners. Begin by choosing a variety of vibrant veggies, including bell peppers, broccoli, and carrots. Cut them into little pieces and combine them with garlic, olive oil, and a small amount of your preferred herbs. Bake them until they become soft and have a hint of caramel. In addition to being visually pleasing, this simple-to-prepare dish is full of vitamins and minerals that are important for a diet that is supportive of prostate cancer.

A bowl of grilled salmon makes a seamless lunchtime addition of lean proteins. Start by marinating salmon fillets in a basic concoction of olive oil, lemon juice, and herbs. The salmon should be grilled to perfection on the grill. Serve it with brown rice or quinoa along with some steamed veggies, such as spinach and asparagus. This hearty bowl delivers omega-3 fatty acids, which support prostate health, in addition to lean protein.

Handheld Choices for Busy Days:

Lunch options that are portable and convenient are essential for maintaining a prostate cancer-friendly diet on busy days. Making wholesome, tasty grab-and-go meals is a great way for beginners to get started.

A Mason jar salad is a simple and convenient lunch idea. Arrange a mix of vibrant veggies, such as cucumbers, cherry tomatoes, and mixed greens, in a Mason jar. Serve with grilled chicken or chickpeas as a source of lean protein, and drizzle with housemade vinaigrette. Before eating, place the jar in the refrigerator and seal it. Even on the busiest days, you can easily acquire vital nutrients with this compact salad.

A thermos-sealed vegetable and lentil soup is a great option for individuals who want something warm. Make a pot of hearty lentil and vegetable soup by combining ingredients such as lentils, tomatoes, celery, and carrots. Transfer the soup into a thermos for a convenient, warm, and satisfying midday meal. This alternative offers a satisfying and substantial meal for people on the go, while also supporting a diet that prevents prostate cancer.

Making a meal that is suitable for a prostate cancer diet doesn't have to be difficult, therefore. These useful, step-by-step recipes offer simplicity without sacrificing flavor or nutritional content, making them suitable for inexperienced cooks. These lunch options, which range from a quick quinoa salad to a veggie-packed sandwich or a portable Mason jar salad, are meant to make following a prostate cancer diet fun and easy for everyone, even on the busiest days.

CHAPTER NINE

FILLING SUPPERTIME RECIPES

Healthy Dinner Choices for the Prostate:

An essential part of a diet for prostate cancer prevention is a well-balanced meal, which supports the unique nutritional requirements related to prostate health while also enhancing general health. Incorporate a range of foods high in nutrients, such as vitamins and minerals, to start. Lean protein sources are better for you since they include less saturated fat, which is good for your prostate. Examples of these include skinless chicken, fish, and tofu. To give a consistent energy release and support general well-being, consume whole grains like quinoa, brown rice, and whole wheat pasta.

Aim for a rainbow of colors with your meal by adding a good helping of vibrant veggies. Broccoli, cauliflower, kale, and spinach are among the many vegetables high in antioxidants that have been associated with a decreased risk of prostate cancer.

Tomatoes also contain lycopene, a potent antioxidant with possible advantages for prostate health. Portion control is essential to guarantee a well-balanced dinner.

Reduce the size of your plates to help control portion sizes and avoid overindulging, which can lead to weight gain and is linked to a higher risk of prostate cancer.

Try enhancing flavor with different herbs and spices instead of relying too much on salt or bad fats. Turmeric, rosemary, thyme, and garlic not only give your food depth, but they may also be good for you. To preserve their nutritious content, cook your meats using healthy techniques like grilling, baking, or steaming.

By emphasizing a well-balanced dinner, you are fostering general well-being via a varied and nourishing meal, in addition to boosting prostate health.

Innovative Methods for Including Lean Meats and Vegetables:

Incorporating creativity into meal preparation is essential for prostate cancer diet followers to maintain interest and provide a diverse range of nutrients. Think of inventive ways to use lean meats and veggies to enhance the meal experience.

To begin, try experimenting with vibrant, unconventional salads. Combine leafy greens, cucumbers, bell peppers, and cherry tomatoes to create a colorful, antioxidant-rich salad. For lean protein, include grilled chicken or salmon to make a filling and prostate-friendly dinner.

Discover the world of pasta substitutes made from vegetables, such as spaghetti squash or zucchini noodles. These low-carb choices deliver more vitamins and minerals along with fewer calories.

Try stir-frying a mix of vegetables with lean meat or tofu for a filling and prostate-healthy meal.

This could be an enjoyable and healthy supper choice because of the blend of flavors and textures.

Use a range of veggies and lean proteins to create interesting wraps and bowls. To increase fiber and support digestive health, choose brown rice bowls or wraps made of whole grains. Use savory marinades and sauces created with herbs, spices, and nutritious oils to add flavor to your food without sacrificing nutrition. You may make delicious and prostate-friendly dishes by experimenting with different cooking techniques and using your imagination.

Delicious and Filling Evening Snacks:

A prostate cancer diet that is both savory and gratifying for evening meals requires careful item selection and expert preparation. To start, choose fresh, high-quality foods to use as the base for your meals. You may add taste to lean proteins like fish, turkey, or grilled chicken without using a lot of salt or toxic additives by seasoning them with a mixture of herbs and spices.

Try a variety of cooking methods to improve the flavor of your food. Vegetables are naturally sweet when roasted, and meats take on a wonderful sear and smoky flavor when grilled.

To enhance the flavor and texture of your food, try adding different textures and tastes. For example, adding crunch and richness to a salad can be achieved by pairing creamy avocado with crunchy almonds or seeds.

Discover the world of spices and herbs to improve the flavor of your dinners at night. Toss salads or main meals with a burst of freshness from fresh basil, cilantro, and mint.

In addition to adding a warming, earthy flavor, turmeric, and ginger may have anti-inflammatory properties. Try a few different combinations and don't be scared to see what works best for your tastes.

If you want your evening meals to be more satisfying, think about adding complex carbohydrates like brown rice, quinoa, or sweet potatoes.

These options contribute to the overall balance of your diet for prostate cancer while also offering long-lasting energy.

You may make tasty, filling dinners that fit within a diet that is prostate-healthy by using different cooking methods, experimenting with herbs and spices, and paying attention to the quality of the components.

CHAPTER TEN

PROSTATE HEALTH THROUGH SMART SNACKING

Ideas for Healthy Snacks to Stop Cravings:

Making wise snack choices is essential to eating a prostate-friendly diet, and discovering nutritious snack substitutes can be fulfilling and good for your general health. It's critical to select snacks that not only satisfy your appetite but also improve the health of your prostate when attempting to minimize urges. Making nutrient-dense food choices is essential to making sure your body is getting the vitamins and minerals it needs.

Start by expanding your snack options to include a range of vibrant fruits and veggies. Antioxidants, which are abundant in these healthful options, are essential for shielding your cells from harm. Carrot sticks and hummus or sliced apples with a smear of almond butter are two easy but tasty options that have a nice crunch and are packed with nutrition. These snacks also contain a lot of fiber, which helps regulate weight and supports digestive health.

Including nuts and seeds in your diet is another shrewd snacking tactic. Because of their high omega-3 fatty acid content, which has been linked to a lower risk of prostate cancer, almonds, walnuts, and chia seeds are great options. Consider portioning these foods ahead of time into small containers or snack-sized bags to make them easier for beginners to access. In this manner, you'll always have a handy and transportable choice on hand for when hunger hits.

If you have a sweet tooth, go for dark chocolate that has at least 70% cocoa. Flavonoids, which are found in dark chocolate, may offer protection against prostate cancer. Enjoy it as a pleasant and antioxidant-rich treat with a handful of berries. To find a balance between enjoyment and health concerns, pay attention to portion proportions.

Selecting tasty and nutrient-rich snacks is an important part of smart eating for prostate health. You may satiate your appetites and promote prostate health by including a range of vibrant fruits and vegetables, nuts, seeds, and conscious quantities of dark chocolate.

Steer Clear of Processed Snacks:

Processed snacks are dangerous for prostate health since they are frequently loaded with harmful fats, high salt content, and preservatives. Avoiding these foods is essential to keeping up a diet that supports general health. Recognizing and avoiding processed food is an essential first step for anyone new on the path to optimal prostate health.

Giving entire, unprocessed foods priority is one important tactic. They consist of nutritious grains, lean meats, and fresh produce. Selecting these natural, high-nutrient options means you won't be consuming the artificial additives and dangerous preservatives that are frequently present in processed snacks. This change promotes better general nutrition in addition to prostate health.

The ability to read food labels becomes essential while trying to stay away from processed foods. Red flags: ingredients like trans fats, artificial flavors, and high-fructose corn syrup suggest a product might not be the greatest choice for prostate health. When choosing snacks as a beginner, pay attention to items that have identifiable, whole-food components and brief ingredient lists.

Making your snacks at home is another frugal strategy. In this manner, you can make sure that your choices are in line with a prostate-friendly diet and maintain complete control over the components. You may have tasty snacks without sacrificing your health by making easy recipes like yogurt parfaits with fresh fruit or homemade trail mix with nuts and seeds.

Prepare ahead of time by putting pre-cut veggies, fruit slices, and a handful of almonds in a small cooler or snack bag. This planning guarantees that you always have healthy options on hand, which lessens the likelihood that you'll grab processed snacks when hunger strikes without warning.

In conclusion, a key component of a diet for prostate cancer is avoiding processed snacks. N00bs may confidently navigate the snacking landscape and maintain their prostate health by selecting healthy, unprocessed foods, carefully reading labels, making snacks at home, and making a strategy.

Healthy Options for Traveling:

When traveling, it's important to prepare ahead and incorporate portable, nutrient-rich options into your meals to maintain a prostate-friendly diet. As a beginner, you should know how important it is to choose snacks that will help your prostate function as a whole in addition to satisfying your hunger.

Preparing an assortment of grab-and-go options ahead of time is one useful step. You can split out mixed nuts, seeds, and dried fruits into compact containers for convenient snack-sized access on hectic days.

This keeps a nutrient-dense snack on hand so you won't have to turn to less healthful options when things become tight.

Another great option for on-the-go that boosts protein and promotes digestive health is Greek yogurt. Pick an unsweetened, plain yogurt and top it with your preferred fruits or a honey drizzle for sweetness. To separate the yogurt and toppings until you're ready to eat your snack, think about utilizing a portable container with sections.

Including entire fruits in your portable snacks is a simple yet powerful tactic. Bananas, oranges, and apples are simple to carry and don't need much preparation. Combine them with a small portion of cheese or a handful of nuts for a well-rounded and fulfilling snack that promotes prostate health.

If you're more of a savory person, make some handmade veggie sticks and serve them with hummus or guacamole. Along with providing a tasty and filling snack, this combo also includes important nutrients including fiber and healthy fats.

Additionally, purchasing portion-controlled, convenient packaging can make it easier for beginners to munch on the go. Prepackaged amounts of cheese, whole-grain crackers, and sliced chicken or turkey can be combined to make a low-preparation, well-balanced snack.

For this reason, choosing simple, nutrient-dense on-the-go snack selections that fit within a prostate cancer diet requires planning. Novices can easily incorporate prostate-supportive foods into their hectic lives by making grab-and-go snacks, adding Greek yogurt, selecting whole fruits, indulging in homemade vegetable sticks, and using portion-controlled packaging.

CHAPTER ELEVEN

HYDRATION AND PROSTATE HEALTH

Importance of Staying Hydrated:

Not only does drinking enough water help promote prostate health in particular, but it's also essential for overall health maintenance. A walnut-sized gland that is a component of the male reproductive system, the prostate needs enough water to function at its best. Water is necessary for many biological processes, such as the movement of nutrients, the removal of waste, and the control of body temperature. When it comes to prostate health, staying hydrated is beneficial since it removes toxins from the body and keeps dangerous compounds from accumulating that may worsen prostate conditions.

Keeping enough water in your system is especially important for people following a diet plan to prevent prostate cancer. Urine concentrations brought on by dehydration can aggravate symptoms associated with the prostate and irritate the urinary system. Eight 8-ounce glasses, or around two liters, is a typical recommendation for how much water an individual should drink during the day. However, individual needs may differ depending on factors such as age, weight, and activity level.

It takes more than simply drinking water to maintain good hydration; one must also incorporate foods high in water in their diet. This two-pronged strategy provides vital nutrients for general health while also assisting with water requirements. Establishing a regimen that includes drinking plenty of water and eating meals high in water content is crucial when starting a path to focus prostate health through hydration.

The Greatest Drinks for Prostate Health:

An essential part of a prostate cancer diet that maximizes prostate health is choosing the appropriate beverages. Although water is the obvious choice when it comes to staying hydrated, some drinks have extra advantages that can help with prostate health. Antioxidants found in green tea, in particular, called catechins, have been linked to possible protection against prostate cancer. A tasty and nutritious addition to the daily routine can include green tea.

Pomegranate juice is another fantastic option because of its high antioxidant content. According to studies, pomegranate juice may have anti-inflammatory and anti-cancer qualities, which makes it a significant part of a diet that is good for the prostate. Still, it's imperative to choose unadulterated, pure types to prevent needless added sugars that can negate the health advantages.

Herbal teas, like nettle tea, have also drawn interest due to their possible advantages for prostate health. It is thought that nettle tea has anti-inflammatory qualities and can help reduce symptoms related to an enlarged prostate. It's best to speak with a healthcare provider before choosing herbal teas to make sure they suit your specific needs and any underlying medical concerns.

While consuming these drinks, it's important to keep your intake of sugary and caffeinated drinks moderated because too much of either could be harmful to your prostate. Maintaining equilibrium and varying the types of beverages you drink can help you develop a fulfilling and prostate-healthy hydration regimen.

Including Foods High in Water and Herbal Teas:

Herbal teas and foods high in water are useful additions that fit well into everyday meals for anyone following a prostate cancer diet. It doesn't have to be difficult to incorporate herbal teas into daily routines, to start. Start by choosing a premium nettle tea or similar herbal infusion with a reputation for being beneficial to the prostate. Making a cup of herbal tea is a calming and convenient way to include these beneficial ingredients in one's diet.

Including fruits and vegetables with a high water content in your diet is a sensible and fun way to consume foods high in water.

Examples of hydrating foods are watermelon, cucumbers, strawberries, and celery. These meals not only help you stay hydrated overall but also offer vital vitamins and minerals. A quick and tasty method to increase nutritional intake and hydration at the same time is to toss these hydrating items into a colorful and varied salad.

It is best to start small and controllable when introducing herbal teas and foods high in water to help a rookie on their path. Making a colorful fruit salad for a snack or designating a certain time of day to sip herbal tea are two examples of how to make the process more pleasurable and sustainable.

Adding variety to the diet and encouraging prostate health in a realistic and doable way can be achieved by gradually increasing the selection of herbal teas and experimenting with different meals high in water content.

All things considered, a diet for prostate cancer that emphasizes hydration entails realizing how important it is to drink enough water, choosing drinks that promote prostate health, and introducing foods high in water and herbal teas into daily routines. Even beginners can confidently and traverse the path to good prostate health by following these doable and guided steps.

CHAPTER TWELVE

LIFESTYLE SUGGESTIONS FOR HEALTHY PROSTATES

Including Exercise in Your Daily Routine:

Starting a road toward the best possible prostate health requires adding exercise to your daily schedule. This need not entail demanding exercise regimens or long gym sessions. Beginners need to begin with easy workouts and build up their intensity gradually. Start by taking 30 minutes a day, at least five days a week, to jog or walk quickly. This low-impact workout helps maintain a healthy weight, which is important for prostate health in addition to enhancing general well-being.

Gradually introduce resistance training with an emphasis on pelvic floor movements and core muscles. These exercises, such as Kegels, improve prostate health in addition to improving bladder control.

Active pursuits like swimming, cycling, or even yoga can be fun substitutes for beginners and provide a comprehensive approach to physical health.

Maintaining consistency is essential. For beginners, the adjustment can be made easy by creating a regular workout schedule and progressively increasing the duration and intensity. Long-term benefits for prostate health can be ensured by scheduling activities and selecting activities that meet personal tastes, which will also make the process pleasurable and sustainable.

Techniques for Stress Management:

Reducing stress is essential to keeping the prostate healthy. Novices might experiment with several stress-reduction strategies that fit their lifestyle. Mindfulness meditation is a great place to start because it provides a simple and efficient way to lower stress. Start with brief sessions that concentrate on breath awareness, and as comfort and confidence increase, progressively increase the duration.

For beginners managing stress, incorporating relaxation techniques like progressive muscle relaxation or deep breathing exercises can be helpful. Creating a calm atmosphere, whether with relaxing music or time spent in nature, offers even more stress reduction. Novices can reduce stress in their daily lives by practicing time management, setting realistic objectives, and learning to prioritize work. These are practical skills.

Exercises that mix mindfulness and physical movement, like yoga and tai chi, are great ways to manage stress. To ease into these activities, beginners can look at online lessons or classes. Including these methods in daily life, even for brief periods at first, can have a substantial effect on stress levels and support prostate health in general.

The Significance of Sufficient Sleep for Prostate Health

For beginners looking to improve the health of their prostate, they must comprehend the importance of getting enough sleep. The first step is to set a regular sleep routine. Try to get between seven and nine hours of good sleep every night to give your body the time it needs to heal and regenerate.

Ensuring a sleep-friendly atmosphere is just as crucial. To encourage sound sleep, novices might make sure their bedroom is cool, quiet, and dark. Reducing screen time before bed and engaging in relaxation exercises like light stretching or reading will help you wind down and get a good night's sleep.

If a sleep disturbance exists, treating it is crucial for the best possible prostate health. To treat conditions like sleep apnea or insomnia, novices should consult a specialist. For beginners, establishing a pre-sleep regimen that includes avoiding coffee and large meals before bedtime helps them develop healthy sleep patterns. Prostate health and general well-being are directly impacted by sleep patterns' consistency and quality. Novices can make a big contribution to maintaining overall energy and a healthy prostate by prioritizing and optimizing sleep.

CHAPTER THIRTEEN

MAINTAINING A LIFESTYLE THAT IS PROSTATE-HEALTHY

Long-Term Tactics To Keep Up A Diet That Is Prostate-Friendly:

A key strategy for improving general prostate health and lowering the risk of prostate cancer is to adopt a diet that is friendly to the prostate. Making reasonable and sustained dietary adjustments is a key component of long-term plans. Start by including a range of vibrant fruits and vegetables in your regular meals. They support prostate health since they are high in vital minerals and antioxidants. Try to get a variety of foods, such as leafy greens, berries, broccoli, and tomatoes.

Make whole grains a mainstay in your diet, along with fruits and vegetables. Good sources of fiber include whole wheat bread, quinoa, and brown rice.

Fiber improves hormone balance and aids in digestion, all of which are beneficial to prostate health.

It might also be advantageous to incorporate healthy fats from foods like olive oil, almonds, and seeds. The omega-3 fatty acids found in these lipids are well-known for their ability to reduce inflammation.

Limit the amount of red and processed meats you eat because research indicates a link between these foods' excessive consumption and a higher risk of prostate cancer. Lean protein options to consider include fish, poultry, tofu, and lentils.

Additionally, restrict your consumption of trans and saturated fats, which are frequently included in processed and fried foods. Instead, to promote the health of your prostate, choose heart-healthy, lean options.

Staying hydrated is essential for sticking to a diet that is good for the prostate. Make sure you consume enough water throughout the day to support your body's overall processes and to help flush out pollutants.

Due to their antioxidant qualities, herbal teas—green tea in particular—are also advised.

The secret to these dietary modifications' success is to stick to them steadily and gradually. To keep organized and guarantee that you are getting a balanced intake of all the necessary nutrients, think about making a weekly meal plan. Accept these food changes as a constructive lifestyle modification for long-term prostate health rather than as restrictive measures.

Frequent Examinations And Observation:

Preventive care for prostate health starts with routine examinations and surveillance. Setting up a schedule for frequent check-ups is crucial for newcomers navigating the healthcare system. Make an appointment with a medical expert, such as a urologist or primary care physician, once a year to talk about your general health, which includes the health of your prostate. It's critical to create an environment of open communication and comfort when addressing any worries or symptoms.

Recognize the significance of regular screenings, such as the digital rectal examination (DRE) and the prostate-specific antigen (PSA) blood test. By identifying any anomalies or indications of prostate problems early on, these exams improve the likelihood that therapy will be effective. To ease any nervousness, it's helpful for beginners to familiarize themselves with the goal and process of these tests.

Note down your family's medical history because prostate health might be influenced by heredity. Share this information with your healthcare practitioner so that they are fully aware of any possible risk factors. As they can affect prostate health, novices should actively participate in conversations about lifestyle issues, such as diet, exercise, and stress management.

An empowering part of long-term prostate care is keeping an eye on your health. Keep an eye out for any changes in sexual function, urination patterns, or general health. Maintain a health notebook to record symptoms or worries; this might be helpful when visiting doctors.

Keep in mind that when it comes to routine checkups, consistency is essential. Include these appointments in your yearly health schedule, and think about setting up alerts to help you remember important checks. Incorporating regular healthcare into your life is a proactive measure toward preserving ideal prostate health.

Honoring Accomplishments And Ongoing Development:

Recognizing accomplishments in living a prostate-friendly lifestyle is crucial for encouraging and reinforcing healthy behaviors. Beginners need to celebrate every little accomplishment along the road. Celebrate and acknowledge your accomplishments, whether they involve regularly going to annual physicals or effectively adding more fruits and vegetables to your diet.

Set attainable objectives and benchmarks for your road toward better prostate health. To increase the tangible and doable nature of your progress, break down larger goals into smaller, more manageable milestones. With each goal accomplished, this strategy prevents beginners from feeling overwhelmed and fosters a sense of success.

Tell someone who can help you succeed—friends, family, or an online prostate health community—about your accomplishments. Making connections with people who have similar objectives to yours can bring support, guidance, and a feeling of unity. Knowing they are not traveling alone might provide novices with drive and comfort.

A key component of keeping up a lifestyle that is prostate-friendly is continuous development. Evaluate your entire lifestyle choices, exercise regimen, and food habits regularly. Look for ways to improve and expand, adjusting to fresh data and investigations into the health of the prostate.

Try out new foods, investigate various exercise regimens, and keep up with developments in prostate health. Adopt a mindset of continuous learning and progress as a rookie. To be informed about the most recent guidelines for prostate health, participate in workshops or seminars, read reliable sources, and communicate with medical professionals.

Novices can create an approach to prostate health that is both sustainable and progressive by acknowledging their accomplishments and embracing ongoing improvement. This optimistic outlook encourages flexibility and resilience, guaranteeing that your efforts will produce long-term advantages for general well-being.

MY GRATITUDES

Dear Valued Readers and Supporters,

I hope this message finds you well. I am writing to express my deepest gratitude to both God and each one of you for the overwhelming support and positive response to my book. Your encouragement and enthusiasm have truly touched my heart, and I am immensely thankful for the journey we are on together.

I believe that every success is a result of collaboration and support from various sources. First and foremost, I want to acknowledge the divine guidance and inspiration that led me to create this cookbook. Without the grace of God, this endeavor would not have been possible.

To my cherished readers, your commitment to exploring healthier dietary options for managing your crises has been both inspiring and humbling.

Your trust in this book" means the world to me, and I am honored to be part of your journey toward improved health and well-being.

Also, I am reaching out to kindly request your valuable feedback on this book. Your thoughts and insights are crucial in helping me enhance and serve you better, ensuring that it continues to meet your needs effectively. Please take a moment to share your thoughts by rating and writing reviews on platforms where the book is available.

Your reviews not only provide me with invaluable feedback but also play a significant role in assisting others in making informed choices. By sharing your experiences, you contribute to a community that values health and wellness, creating a positive impact on countless lives.

Additionally, I encourage you to share this book with your friends, family and loved ones. Together, we can extend the reach of this promising resource, offering support and guidance to those who may benefit from it.

Having this knowledge and seeking medical advice from your specialist I anticipate a turnaround for us.

Once again, thank you from the depths of my heart for your unwavering support. I am committed to continually improving and serving you better. Let us continue this journey together, promoting health, well-being, and a shared sense of community.

With sincere appreciation,

[Emmy Brooks]

Author, "PROSTATE CANCER DIET COOKBOOK"

www.ingramcontent.com/pod-product-compliance
Lightning Source LLC
Chambersburg PA
CBHW050930260726
48660CB00001B/488